THE NEW SUGAR BUSTERS!®

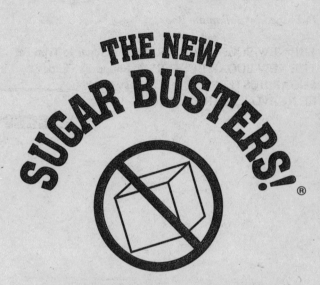

SHOPPER'S GUIDE

Published by Ballantine Books:

THE NEW SUGAR BUSTERS!®: Cut Sugar to Trim Fat
THE NEW SUGAR BUSTERS!®: Shopper's Guide
SUGAR BUSTERS!®: Quick & Easy Cookbook
EL NUEVO SUGAR BUSTERS!®

Books published by The Random House Publishing Group
are available at quantity discounts on bulk purchases for
premium, educational, fund-raising, and special sales use.
For details, please call 1-800-733-3000.

THE NEW SUGAR BUSTERS!®

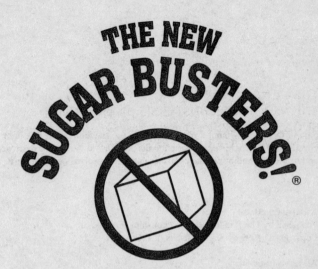

SHOPPER'S GUIDE

H. LEIGHTON STEWARD
MORRISON C. BETHEA, M.D.
SAMUEL S. ANDREWS, M.D.
LUIS A. BALART, M.D.

BALLANTINE BOOKS • NEW YORK

Sale of this book without a front cover may be unauthorized. If this book is coverless, it may have been reported to the publisher as "unsold or destroyed" and neither the author nor the publisher may have received payment for it.

A Ballantine Book
Published by The Random House Publishing Group
Copyright © 1999 by Sugar Busters, L.L.C.

All rights reserved.

Published in the United States by Ballantine Books, an imprint of The Random House Publishing Group, a division of Random House, Inc., New York, and simultaneously in Canada by Random House of Canada Limited, Toronto. Originally published in slightly different form by Ballantine Books, a division of Random House, Inc., in 1999.

SUGAR BUSTERS! is a trademark owned by Sugar Busters, L.L.C. All rights are reserved. This trademark may not be used in any form without express written consent of Sugar Busters, L.L.C.

BALLANTINE and colophon are registered trademarks of Random House, Inc.

ISBN 978-0-345-45922-0

Printed in the United States of America

www.ballantinebooks.com

First Edition: January 1999
First Mass Market Edition: January 2004

OPM   10   9   8   7   6   5

Table of Contents

Contents

Introduction

The authors of *Sugar Busters!: Cut Sugar to Trim Fat* have developed the *Sugar Busters! Shopper's Guide* to help you make better selections in your local grocery store, supermarket, and delicatessen, and how to make better selections when eating out. Many of you have voiced to us frustrations concerning which items are best for you. Grocery shopping is difficult. Advertising and labeling are often misleading and, at best, confusing. That is why we are including a section on reading labels. We, the authors of *Sugar Busters!*, know that our concept is valid, but, if you do not know how to make correct choices regarding what you eat, *Sugar Busters!* may not work for you. Therefore, we have developed this guide to help you succeed on *Sugar Busters!*

Sugar Busters! also has introduced its own products in categories where we feel there is the greatest demand. We have done this to ensure the availability of "legal " (acceptable) products as well as to protect the integrity of our concept. The authors have personally participated in the formulation of the products regarding ingredients and also to ensure that the foods are of excellent taste as measured by anyone's standards. Many of the products are available in your local area, but if not, please ask your grocery store manager to contact Boudreaux Foods in New Orleans, Louisiana, at www.sugarbusterfood.com, who will try to make these products available in your local market.

In October 2003, the RAND Corporation reported that the number of people at least 100 pounds overweight had quadrupled since the 1980s. Do not become one of these high-risk people. *Sugar Busters!*® can help you achieve this goal. The *Sugar Busters!* glycemic index or load approach for choosing the best carbohydrates has now been supported by the World Health Organization as well as many professional nutritionists.

The *Sugar Busters!* lifestyle is logical, practical, and reasonable. It does *not* involve weighing, measuring, or counting, but it does involve making better choices about what you eat, and it does involve moderation, especially in portion sizes. If you make healthy and nutritious choices and your servings of these choices are moderate, there is no need to worry about counting calories, which, in most instances, would be inaccurate and not even beneficial to what you are trying to achieve. *Sugar Busters!* is about lean and trimmed meats, high-fiber vegetables, whole grains, nuts, most fruits, and, if you choose, alcohol responsibly and in moderation.

Sugar Busters! is very careful and concerned about too much fat, especially saturated fat. This can be animal as well as trans-fats, which are hydrogenated or partially hydrogenated vegetable oils that are frequently added to grocery products or used in commercial fast-food kitchens. On *Sugar Busters!* you generally will be eating 40 percent (or slightly more) carbohydrates, 30 percent protein, and 30 percent fat, only 10 percent of which should be saturated fat. These parameters are perfectly healthy and conform to those recommended by the American Heart Association. There are only a few common foods that you should avoid, such as white or red potatoes, beets, corn and corn products, white flour products, white rice, carrots, and a few of the higher glycemic fruits, such as ripe bananas and raisins.

You will notice when shopping for *Sugar Busters!* items that your best choices are around the perimeter of the store rather than in the center, where the processed foods are located. In making your choices, try to select those products that have as little refined sugar as possible, preferably no more than three grams of added refined sugar per serving. Always remember that fresh is best, then frozen, and canned is often the least desirable. Different brands of the same food often vary considerably in the added ingredients. Therefore, reading labels until you are familiar with those items that are best for you will really help in cutting sugar.

Sugar Busters! highly recommends exercise. Unfortunately, over 70 percent of you do not and will not exercise, but you can still improve your weight and health by following the *Sugar Busters!* nutritional lifestyle.

What will *Sugar Busters!* do for you? It will help you achieve your ideal body weight (genetically pre-determined), reduce your risks of diabetes and hypertension, and slow the aging of your blood vessels, as well as help prevent many other obesity-related health problems. If you are diabetic, *Sugar Busters!* will make it much easier to control your blood sugars. Those of you who suffer from hypoglycemia (low blood sugar) will also benefit from the *Sugar Busters!* lifestyle.

How is all of this achieved on *Sugar Busters!*? By eating in a healthy and nutritious fashion and by making better carbohydrate choices, you can go through the day with lower insulin levels. You cannot live without insulin, but you can live much better without too much insulin. Insulin, in addition to transporting glucose into cells for some of our energy needs, also makes you store sugar and fat as fat, prevents you from burning fat efficiently, and instructs your liver to produce additional amounts of cholesterol. Simply stated, higher than normal levels of insulin make us fat and flabby and our blood vessels age more quickly. This is something that we all would like to avoid, and the *Sugar Busters!* lifestyle will help you achieve this goal.

Try *Sugar Busters!* You will like it. You will look and feel your best. It does not involve any costly supplements or additives but *only* involves making good, nutritious decisions about what you eat. This shopper's guide will help you get on your way. In addition, we have added a section on how to eat out successfully on *Sugar Busters!*

Enjoy and *bon appétit!*

THE NEW
SUGAR BUSTERS!®

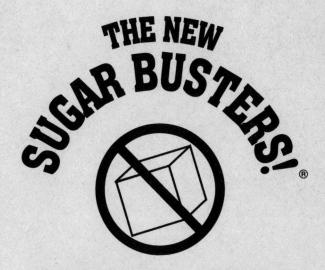

SHOPPER'S GUIDE

The Food Lists

What follows is a list of the various foods, grouped according to where they are generally found in the store. But first, here are a few over-all tips on interpreting some things that might confuse you. For instance, when you pick up a can of boiled tomatoes and see that the listed ingredients are simply tomatoes and salt, yet the standard chart reads four grams of sugar, you should realize that tomatoes are really a fruit and, as such, must have their fructose content listed as sugar. This does not mean you should avoid boiled tomatoes! Remember, natural fructose is a good source of sugar and is not bad for you unless it has been concentrated, as in high fructose corn syrup, or consumed in large quantities with other sugars or saturated fats during the same meal. The same goes for peanut butter, as long as there has been no sugar added.

1

Since cooking raises the glycemic index—or blood-sugar-elevating effect—of carbohydrates, you can understand why it is better to replace most canned carbohydrates (except for green leafy vegetables) with the fresh, dried, or frozen variety.

When you prepare your dried beans, fresh vegetables, whole-grain pasta, or brown rice, do not overcook them. Instead, cook them al dente, or just a little bit firm. This will ensure a lower glycemic effect. Remember that your ancient ancestors actually ate their grains and vegetables completely raw—and obviously it worked just fine, otherwise we wouldn't be here today!

Finally, one last reminder so you will not have to count and measure: eat three platefuls a day with only appropriate snacks in between. A green salad on the side is all right. Do not cheat while you are trying to lose weight, but once you have achieved that goal, treat yourself occasionally to something that suits your fancy. But remember—too many treats will mean more fat on you!

The following lists will range from those containing some common brand names to simply a general statement, for example, that all unsweetened, no-sugar-added pickles are okay.

FRESH PRODUCE DEPARTMENT

VEGETABLES

Artichokes
Arugula
Asparagus

Bean sprouts
Bell pepper (red and green)
Bok choy
Broccoli
Brussels sprouts

Cabbage
Cauliflower
Celery
Cucumber
Eggplant
Endive

Vegetables

Leeks
Lettuce

Mushrooms
Mustard greens

Okra
Onion—white, red, yellow

Peas
Pumpkin

Radicchio
Radishes

Sauerkraut
Snow peas
Spinach
Squash—yellow, butternut, spaghetti,
    acorn
String beans

Sweet potatoes/yams (in moderation)

Tofu
Tomatoes
Turnip greens

Vegetables

Watercress

Zucchini

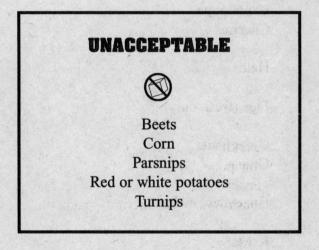

UNACCEPTABLE

Beets
Corn
Parsnips
Red or white potatoes
Turnips

FRUITS

      Apples
      Apricots
      Avocados

      Blackberries
      Blueberries
      Boysenberries

      Canteloupe
      Cherries

      Dates

      Figs (fresh only)

      Grapefruits
      Grapes

      Honeydew melon

      Kiwis

      Lemons
      Limes

      Mandarin oranges
      Musk melons

Fruits

Nectarines

Oranges

Peaches
Pears
Persimmons
Plums
Pomegranates

Raspberries

Satsumas
Strawberries

Tangerines

UNACCEPTABLE

Bananas (ripe)
Pineapples
Raisins
Large servings of watermelon

MEAT DEPARTMENT
&
REFRIGERATED ITEMS

Alligator
Antelope

Bacon (preferably not sugar cured)
Beef (lean and trimmed)

Canadian bacon
Chicken

Dove
Duck

Elk

Goose

Ham (if not sugar cured)
Hamburger (preferably lean)

Lamb

Ostrich

Partridge
Pheasant
Pork

Quail

Rabbit

Turkey

Veal
Venison

UNACCEPTABLE

Cuts of beef & lamb containing
marbled fat
Cold cuts with dextrose or other
added sugars
Fatty bacon

DAIRY DEPARTMENT

Butter

Cheese
Cottage cheese
Cream

Dannon Light Yogurt with aspartame

Egg Beaters™
Eggs

Milk—2% or less fat preferred

Non-hydrogenated margarine or butter
    substitutes

Philadelphia® Cream Cheese
    (preferably light or low fat)

Dairy Department

Sour cream (preferably light
or low fat)

Yogurt, no-sugar-added yogurts like
Mountain High® Original Style
Plain
Mountain High® Original Style
Vanilla

SEAFOOD DEPARTMENT

Alaskan pollock

Blue crab

Carp
Catfish
Clams (raw)
Cod
Cobia
Crawfish

Dolphin
Drum
Dungeness crab

Eel

Flounder

Seafood Department

Grouper

Haddock
Halibut
Herring

King crab

Lobster

Mahi-Mahi
Monkfish
Mussels

Octopus
Orange roughy
Oysters

Perch
Pike
Pompano

Redfish

Salmon
Scallops
Sea bass
Shrimp

Seafood Department

Snails
Snapper
Snow crab
Sole
Stone crab

Tilapia
Trout
Tuna

Whitefish

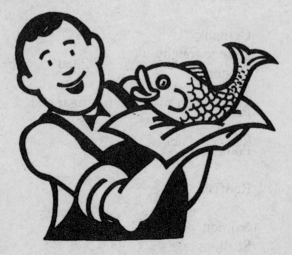

DELI

Cheeses, in moderation
Cole Slaw, if no sugar added

Fruit salad, if no sugar added

Green bean salad, if no sugar added

All meats with no sugar added

Mixed bean salads, if no sugar added

Roasted chicken

Tomato & cucumber salads,
      etc., if no sugar added

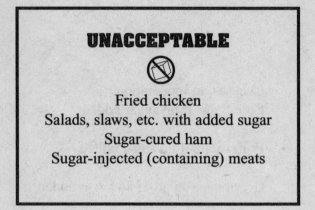

UNACCEPTABLE

Fried chicken
Salads, slaws, etc. with added sugar
Sugar-cured ham
Sugar-injected (containing) meats

BAKERY/BREADS

Beware of added sugars and breads that are not 100 percent whole grain or 100 percent whole wheat.

Sugar Busters!® French Bread/Po-Boy
Sugar Busters!® Dinner Rolls
Sugar Busters!® Pistolettes
Sugar Busters!® Pita Bread
Sugar Busters!® Multigrain
Sugar Busters!® Rustic Loaf
Sugar Busters!® Baguette
Sugar Busters!® Sliced Stone Ground
        Whole Wheat Bread
Sugar Busters!® Sliced Multigrain Onion
        Bread
Sugar Busters!® Sliced Flaxseed Bread

The Baker Pumpernickel
The Baker Sunflower Rye
The Baker Whole Grain Rye
The Baker Whole Wheat

Bakery/Breads

Damascus Bakeries Whole
    Wheat Pita

Food For Life Ezekiel 4:9™ Sprouted
    Grain Bread
Food For Life Ezekiel 4:9™ Sesame
    Sprouted Grain Bread
Food For Life Ezekiel 4:9™ Sprouted
    Grain Hot Dog Buns
Food For Life Ezekiel 4:9™ Sprouted
    Grain Burger Buns
Food For Life Ezekiel 4:9™ Sprouted
    Grain Tortillas

Mestemacher Organic Four Grain Bread
Mestemacher Organic
    Sunflower Seed Bread
Mestemacher Organic Three Grain Bread
Mestemacher Whole Rye Bread

Pacific Bakery Whole Grain Spelt Bread
Pacific Bakery Multi-Grain Bread
Pacific Bakery Whole-Grain Rye Bread
Pacific Bakery Whole-Grain Kamut
    Bread
Pacific Bakery Whole-Grain Wheat
    Bread

Bakery/Breads

Pacific Bakery Multi-Grain Bread with
Flax Seeds

Toufayan® Oat Bran Pita
Toufayan® Whole Wheat Pita

Whole Foods Seven Grain
Whole Foods Market Organic
Whole Foods Whole Wheat Pita

Whole grain pumpernickel, 100%
Whole grain rye, 100%

Wild's European Style Oatmeal Bread
Wild's Komis Brot
Wild's Westphalian Pumpernickel
Wild's Whole Grain

UNACCEPTABLE

Breads that have sugars added (including
corn syrup, molasses, etc.) or are not stone
ground whole grain breads

BEVERAGES

Caffeine-free diet colas
Coffee
Crystal Light®

Decaf coffee
Diet colas and sodas
Diet ginger ale
Diet root beer
Diet Snapple®
Diet tonic water

Lemonade (with artificial sweetener)

No-sugar-added tea

Sugar Busters!® Refresher sports drink

TAB®

UNACCEPTABLE

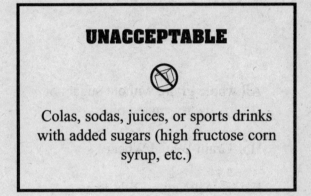

Colas, sodas, juices, or sports drinks
with added sugars (high fructose corn
syrup, etc.)

SNACKS & CRACKERS

All whole grain, without sugars or
hydrogenated oils

Hol-Grain Whole Wheat

Kavli® All Natural Whole
Grain Crispbread
Kavli® Crispy Thin 5 Grain
Kavli® 5 Grain

Manischewitz whole wheat Matzos

Ryvita® crackers (light & dark rye)

Terra® Sweet Potato Chips

Wasa® Fiber Rye
Wasa® Hearty Rye
Wasa® Light Rye

Wasa® Multigrain
Wasa® Organic Rye
Wasa® Soya Crispbread

Whole Foods 365 Baked Woven Wheats
Whole grain wheat wafers

Zapp's Sweet Potato Chips

See also Nuts & Seeds (pages 24–25),
Fruits (pages 6–7),
Vegetables (pages 3–5),
Peanut Butter (pages 35-36),
and Cocoa/Chocolate (pages 37–38),
which can all be used as snacks.

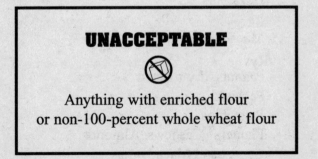

UNACCEPTABLE

Anything with enriched flour
or non-100-percent whole wheat flour

NUTS & SEEDS

All nuts, without added sugar, honey, etc.
Almonds

Brazil nuts

Cashews

Flaxseed (ground)

Hazelnuts

Macadamia nuts

Peanuts, dry roasted
Pecans
Pistachios
Planters® Cashews, Almonds,
      and Macadamias—
      Select Mix

Nuts

Planters® Dry Roasted Pistachios
Planters® Mixed Nuts
Planters® Select Mix
Pumpkin seeds

Sesame seeds
Soy nuts
Sunflower kernels

Walnuts

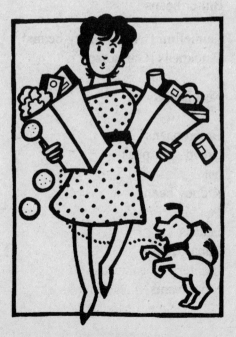

BEANS

Black beans
Black-eyed peas
Butter beans

Cannellini (white kidney beans)
Chickpeas (Garbanzo)

Fava beans

Green beans
Green split peas

Kidney beans

Lentils
Lima beans

Navy beans

Beans

Pink beans
Pinto beans
Purple hull beans

Red beans

Soybeans

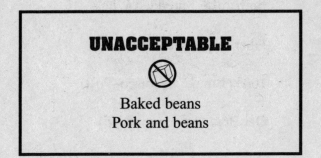

UNACCEPTABLE

Baked beans
Pork and beans

CEREAL

COLD CEREAL
  Barbara's® Breakfast O's
  Barbara's® Shredded Wheat

  Fiber One® (General Mills)

  100% Bran™ (Nabisco, Post)

  Oat Bran (no sugar added)

  Perfect Harvest™ Multigrain Cereal

  Quaker® Unprocessed Bran

  Puffed Kashi Seven Whole Grains &
      Sesame

  Shredded Wheat and Bran
      (Post or Nabisco)

Cold Cereal

Uncle Sam® Cereal

Wheat Montana 7-Grain Cereal

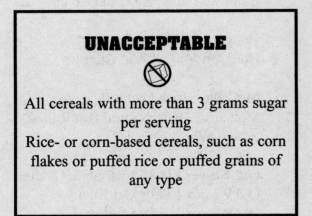

UNACCEPTABLE

All cereals with more than 3 grams sugar per serving
Rice- or corn-based cereals, such as corn flakes or puffed rice or puffed grains of any type

HOT CEREAL

Arrowhead Mills® 7 Grain Cereal

Bob's Red Mill® 5 Grain Rolled Cereal
Bob's Red Mill® 7 Grain Cereal
Bob's Red Mill® 10 Grain Cereal

Hodgson Mill® Oat Bran
Hodgson Mill® Wheat Bran

McCann's® Irish Oatmeal
Mother's® 100% Natural Hot Rolled
        Wheat Cereal

Old Wessex Ltd.™ Irish Style Oatmeal
Old Wessex Ltd.™ Oat Bran
Old Wessex Ltd.™ Scottish Style
        Porridge Oats

Old World Bulgur Organic Wheat

Quaker® Old Fashioned Quaker Oats
Quaker® Barley
Quaker® MultiGrain

UNACCEPTABLE

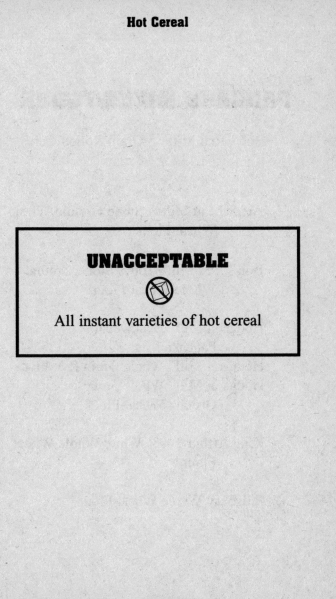

All instant varieties of hot cereal

PANCAKE MIXES/FLOUR

Arrowhead Mills® Stone Ground Whole
    Wheat Flour

Bob's Red Mill® 100% Stone Ground
    Whole Wheat Flour

Hodgson Mill® Buckwheat
    Pancake Mix
Hodgson Mill® Whole Grain Rye Flour
Hodgson Mill® Whole Stone
    Ground Wheat Flour

King Arthur 100% White Whole Wheat
    Flour

Pillsbury Whole Wheat Flour

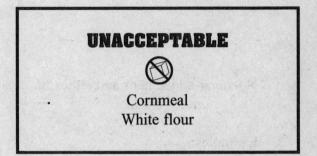

UNACCEPTABLE

Cornmeal
White flour

JAMS/JELLIES

No-sugar-added jams and jellies, in
limited amounts.

Examples:

Dickinson's® Purely Fruit®

Marie Sharp's All Natural Papaya Jam,
Orange, Guava Jam

Polaner® All Fruit®

St. Dalfour 100% Fruit
Smucker's® Simply 100% Fruit®
Sorrell Ridge® 100% Fruit

PEANUT BUTTER

No-sugar-added natural peanut butters

Arrowhead Mills® Peanut Butter
Arrowhead Mills® Almond Butter

Eastwind Cashew Butter

Kettle™ Almond, Cashew, Hazelnut, and
    Sunflower Butters

Krema Natural Peanut Butter

Krinos® Tahini

Laura Scudder's All Natural Peanut
    Butter

Maranatha Almond Butter
Maranatha Cashew Butter

Peanut Butter

Maranatha Raw Tahini
Maranatha Roasted Tahini

Smucker's® Natural

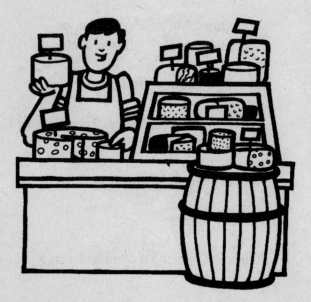

COCOA/CHOCOLATE

All no-sugar-added baking chocolate
All chocolate with more than 60% cocoa,
    in limited amounts

Baker's® Unsweetened Baking
    Chocolate Squares

Carnation® Fat Free Cocoa Mix

Green & Black's Organic Dark
    Chocolate

Guanaja Dark Chocolate

Hershey's® Baking Chocolate,
    unsweetened

Lindt's 70% or 85% Cocoa chocolate bar

Cocoa/Chocolate

Nestlé® unsweetened

Nestlé® Choco-Bake, unsweetened

No-sugar-added candies with less than 10
grams of sugar alcohols (maltitol,
xylitol, sorbitol, etc.) per serving

Rapunzel Bittersweet Chocolate

Valor® Dark Chocolate 70% Cocoa with
Almonds

Valrhona Guanaja 70% Cocoa

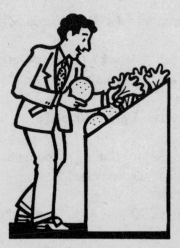

TEA/COFFEE

All decaffeinated coffee & tea

Black teas

Decaffeinated espresso

Green teas

White teas

Limited amounts of caffeinated types

JUICE

All no-sugar-added juices in limited
      amounts
Apple juice

100% cranberry juice

Grape juice (no sugar added)
Grapefruit juice (fresh squeezed, or from
      concentrate, no sugar added) in
     · moderation

Orange juice (fresh squeezed, or from
      concentrate, no sugar added) in
      moderation

Tomato juice

SOUP

CANNED/CONDENSED SOUP

> All with no sugar added and/or white
> flour or potatoes or white rice
> added (which may not be many)

> ShariAnn's Spicy French Green Lentil
> Soup
> ShariAnn's Indian Black Bean and Rice
> Soup

DRY SOUP

> All with no sugar or white flour
> or potatoes or white rice added.
> Examples:

> Amy's Split Pea Soup
> Amy's Vegetable Barley Soup

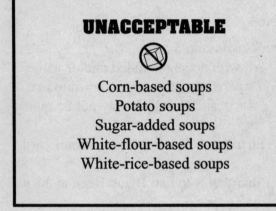

UNACCEPTABLE

Corn-based soups
Potato soups
Sugar-added soups
White-flour-based soups
White-rice-based soups

CANNED MEAT/FISH

All with no sugar added

Chicken in water
Crabmeat

Escargot

Mackerel

Salmon
Sardines
Shrimp

Tuna in water, olive oil, or
        canola oil

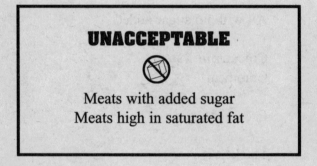

UNACCEPTABLE

Meats with added sugar
Meats high in saturated fat

OLIVES/PICKLES/ GARNISHES

All with no sugar added

Capers
Cocktail onions

Dill pickles (with no sugar added)

Grape leaves

Mt. Olive No Sugar Added Bread &
     Butter Pickles

Olives, all

Pearl onions

Roasted peppers

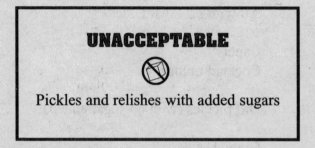

UNACCEPTABLE

Pickles and relishes with added sugars

CONDIMENTS

Hot sauce, all, with no sugar added

Sugar Busters!® Mayonnaise
Mayonnaise (preferably light
     or low fat with no sugar
     added)
Mustards, all, with no sugar added

Vinegar, all

NOTE: Many condiments contain some added sugars but can be consumed in limited quantities. Others, like thick teriyaki sauces, can contain large amounts of sugars and should be avoided.

Coming soon:
    Sugar Busters® Ketchup and
    Bar-B-Que Sauce.

CANNED FRUIT

All "legal" fruits (pages 6–7) with no
sugar added

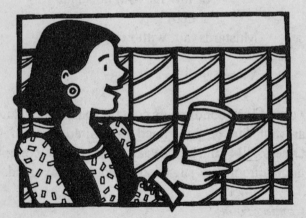

CANNED VEGETABLES

All "legal" vegetables (pages 3–5) with
no sugar added (fresh or
frozen would be better)

Examples:

Hearts of palm

Progresso® Artichoke Hearts
Progresso® Crushed Tomatoes
Progresso® Peeled Tomatoes

Roberts' Big Red Tomatoes,
no salt added
Rotel Diced Tomatoes & Green Chilies

Salsas with no sugar added

Canned Vegetables

Trappey's® Beans—Black-Eyed
Peas, Kidney, Pinto,
White Butter
Trappey's® Jalapeños

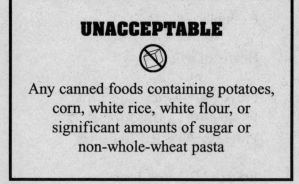

UNACCEPTABLE

Any canned foods containing potatoes,
corn, white rice, white flour, or
significant amounts of sugar or
non-whole-wheat pasta

SALAD DRESSINGS

All with little or no added sugar and no
   partially hydrogenated vegetable
   oils

Examples:

Sugar Busters!® Ranch
Sugar Busters!® Blue Cheese
Sugar Busters!® Caesar
Sugar Busters!® Italian
Sugar Busters!® 1000 Island

Annie's Naturals Caesar

SPAGHETTI SAUCE

All with no sugar or white flour added.

Examples:

Alessi sauces with no sugar added

Bove's of Vermont

Classico® sauces with no sugar added
Colavita® Tomato Sauce, London Style
Cucina Antica™

Enrico's

Garden Valley Sundried Tomato Salsa

Millina's Finest
Mom's Pasta Sauce
Muir Glen® Organic

Rao's Homemade™

Walnut Acres®

Look for Sugar Busters!™ Pasta Sauces
in the future.

PASTA

All 100 percent whole-wheat pastas.

Examples:

Sugar Busters® Stone Ground Whole
     Wheat Pastas: Angel Hair,
     Spaghetti, Fetuccine, Lasagna,
     Spirals, and Egg Noodles

Annie's Organic Whole Wheat Spaghetti
Annie's Organic Whole Wheat Linguini

Bionaturae Whole Wheat Pasta

Capellini (angel hair), in small amounts
Cuore Italiano Durum Wheat Semolina

DeBoles® Whole Wheat Pasta

Pasta

Eden® Organic Golden Amber
 Durum Wheat

Farro Grain Bio Natural Whole Durum
 Wheat
Farro Grain VitaSpelt Whole Grain Spelt
 Pasta

Hodgson Mill® Whole Wheat Fettucine
Hodgson Mill® Whole Wheat, Whole
 Grain Spaghetti
Hodgson Mill® Whole Wheat
 Spinach Spaghetti

Whole Foods 365 Organic Whole Wheat
 Penne Rigate

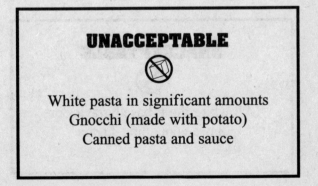

UNACCEPTABLE

White pasta in significant amounts
Gnocchi (made with potato)
Canned pasta and sauce

GRAVY

All natural, no-sugar-or-white-flour-added gravies. Also beware of the addition of maltodextrin and cornstarch.

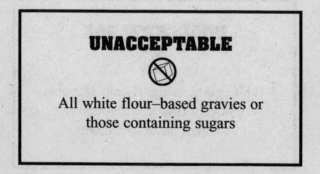

UNACCEPTABLE

All white flour–based gravies or those containing sugars

BOX DINNERS/
PREPARED FOODS

All without added sugars, white flour
products, white rice, white
potatoes, or corn

Examples:

Fantastic Foods® Semolina Couscous

Hodgson Mill® Whole Wheat
Macaroni & Cheese

Tofu Burger
Tofu Scrambler

ETHNIC/SPECIALTY FOODS

Abraham's Hummus

Bamboo shoots
Bean threads (Chinese
        cellophane noodles)
Bok choy

Cedar's® Taboule

Fantastic Foods® Hummus

Guacamole

Hot Mama's Hummus
Hummus in general

Salsa
Snow peas

Soy sauce

Tabbouleh in general
Tofu
Tofu Burger
Tofu Scramble

Water chestnuts
Whole wheat couscous in general
Whole wheat pita bread (see
        Bakery/Breads)
Whole wheat tortillas in general

UNACCEPTABLE

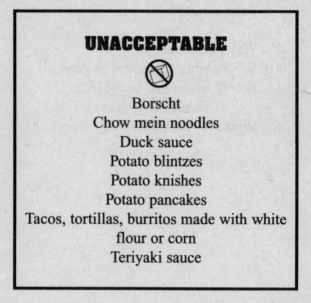

Borscht
Chow mein noodles
Duck sauce
Potato blintzes
Potato knishes
Potato pancakes
Tacos, tortillas, burritos made with white
flour or corn
Teriyaki sauce

RICE

Brown basmati rice
Brown rice (not instant)

Hadden House Extra Fancy
     Cultivated Wild Rice

Kasha

Old World Pilaf

Texmati® Basmati Brown Rice
Toasted almond pilaf

Wild rice

Zatarain's® Brown Rice
     Jambalaya Mix

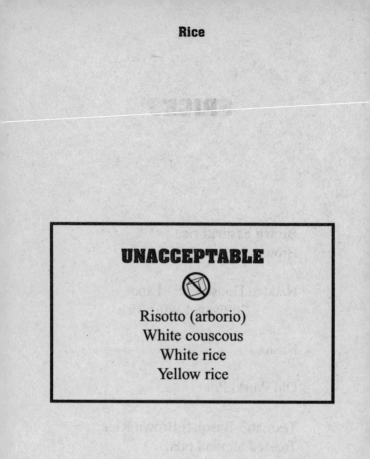

UNACCEPTABLE

Risotto (arborio)
White couscous
White rice
Yellow rice

SPICES

All with no significant amount of added sugar, or that will be used only in significant quantities (which means nearly all spices are "legal")

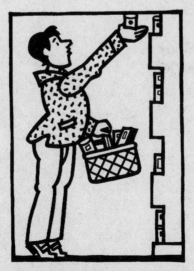

COOKING OIL

Canola
Corn

Olive

PAM®
Peanut

Safflower
Sunflower

CAKE/FLOUR

Stone ground whole wheat flours

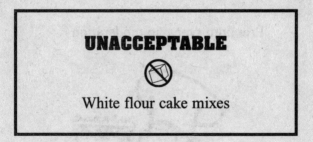

UNACCEPTABLE

White flour cake mixes

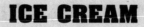

No sugar added ice creams

Sugar Busters!® Vanilla, Chocolate,
Strawberry, and Butter Pecan
ice creams

Premium types, in moderation

FROZEN FOOD

All "legal" vegetables on pages 3–5
and all using same criteria as
          prepared foods

Examples:

Boca® Burgers

Gardenburgers®
Gorton's® Grilled Fish Fillets—
          Lemon Pepper

Mrs. Paul's® Fish Fillets—
          Lemon Pepper
Mrs. Paul's® Grilled Fish
          Fillets
Mrs. Paul's® Grilled Salmon—
          Creamy Dill

ALCOHOL

First choice, dry red wines
White wines
Grain alcohols (scotch, bourbon,
      rye, etc.)
Rum
Tequila
Vodka

UNACCEPTABLE

Beer
Sweet after-dinner wines, i.e. port,
sweet sauternes, any hard liquors with
mixers containing added sugars

Tips for
Lite-Weight Travel

Excess poundage, whether in your bags or around your middle, can make either business or personal travel a lot less comfortable. While many of us have figured out how to lighten our loads by choosing a few garments that mix and match well, most of us seem to be less creative when confronted with the menus placed before us in restaurants across the country. Statistics show that we increase our risk for health problems as our body weight reaches obesity levels (twenty percent or more overweight). This should be incentive enough for us to learn how to make better choices now that the secret is out that it's primarily refined sugar and a handful of carbohydrates that cause the storage of most of our body fat.

Sugar can become body fat? Absolutely; it is explicitly stated in Arthur C. Guyton's *Textbook of Medical Physiology*. That's why we need to know how to bargain for alternatives when we are at the mercy of a menu and a waiter in places far from home.

The first, and usually the hardest, choice presents itself when a basket of warm, white, and probably fiberless bread is placed right under your nose. Beside it is usually a small bowl or a few pats of fresh butter. Bread smells great, you are hungry because it is mealtime, and your mouth begins to water. But first, you should ask for whole-grain or dark bread; they just might have it. Such substitutions are becoming commonplace, even in French-bread cities like New Orleans, Louisiana. It has been requested enough by the followers of the *Sugar Busters!* lifestyle that restaurants have responded favorably and have made healthier breads available.

Breads with a higher percentage of whole grains, while much better for your waistline and general health, still should be eaten *in moderate quantities.* If restaurants just don't have acceptable bread, please resist the temptation to eat the highly refined white types. Making a bad decision at the beginning of a meal often turns into a "what-the-heck" attitude. You have already cheated, so, you could rationalize, you might as well order anything you want. Please don't!

The list of appetizers can be quite limited and

occasionally all may be unacceptable. If none of them is totally acceptable, choose the one that has the least amount of "illegal" ingredients. Also, don't forget to check out the soups, since one might be an excellent substitution for an appetizer.

Ordering the main course is usually easier than trying to satisfy the white-bread or appetizer challenge. Fortunately, most restaurants will allow reasonable substitutions, and the easier you make it for them, the more likely they are to comply. To make it easy for the waiter, scan the vegetables offered with the various entrées and suggest that you would like the green beans from a different entrée instead of the mashed potatoes offered with your preferred entrée. It is difficult for a restaurant to deny you something already being prepared in its kitchen that day.

What do you do if the menu offers only low-fiber, blood-sugar-elevating carbohydrates like potatoes, corn, white rice, and white pasta? Don't give up! Good restaurants like to please you. Instead, ask for a grilled tomato or sautéed vegetables. If they cannot accommodate you, just eat the smallest amount of high-insulin-producing carbohydrates to get you through the meal.

If the sauce being served with your pork chop

is of a sweet variety, ask for it in a small dish on the side. That way, if your pork chop is cooked too dry, you can dab each bite of meat in the sauce instead of "pigging out" on a large amount of the sauce. As with substitutions for vegetables, check out other sauces being served and see if a low-sugar sauce is available.

Another tough decision comes when everyone at the table orders some sugary dessert and you don't want to sit there with an empty plate. If you have been moderate with your main meal, order some high-fiber berries like raspberries or strawberries topped with a little real cream and, if you must, sprinkle them with your favorite artificial sweetener. Or ask for a wedge of cheese, a cup of decaffeinated cappuccino, or, as the Europeans do, finish your meal with a green salad with a tasty sugar-free dressing.

If you are with a business guest and don't want to make your client feel self-conscious, simply order vanilla ice cream. While not ideal, most premium vanilla ice creams served in good restaurants contain only moderate amounts of sugar. If the restaurant doesn't have vanilla ice cream, you have at least tried to join your companion in a normal dessert and they won't think you are some strange, antisocial individual. The worst thing you can do is end a great *Sugar Busters!* meal by giving in and eating a big sugary dessert and storing not only the sugar as body fat but increasing the problems that can occur when elevated insulin levels are present with any saturated fat you might have consumed with the rest of your meal.

Try these recommendations. You won't always succeed in getting what you wish, but if we all keep asking, more and better choices will appear. They are already showing up in restaurants and groceries across the country, and the expansion of choices should continue. It is very difficult to resist temptation when the choices are extremely limited or nonexistent, but again, keep asking and maybe someday even airline snacks or meals will change. Good luck and happy traveling and dining.

Reading Labels

Federal regulations require that food and beverage producers print certain "nutritional facts" on their product labels. Frequently, these facts are confusing and even misleading to the consumer. In an effort to help you better understand labeling and to make you a better *Sugar Busters!* shopper, we have included this section on reading labels.

Nutritional facts are based on a single recommended serving size. The information provided usually pertains to calories, total fats, carbohydrates, proteins, cholesterol, vitamins, minerals, and "other ingredients." We will discuss each one of these items separately so you can understand their significance.

The listed "serving size" may or may not be applicable, depending on what *your* average ser-

Reading Labels

EXAMPLES OF NUTRITIONAL LABELS

Sugar Busters!®
Acceptable

Sugar Busters!®
Unacceptable

Nutrition Facts

Serving Size ⅙ cup (199g)
Servings Per Container 2½

Amount Per Serving

Calories 20   Calories from Fat 0

	% Daily Value*
Total Fat 0g	**0%**
Saturated Fat 0g	**0%**
Cholesterol 0mg	**0%**
Sodium 420mg	**17%**
Total Carbohydrate 3g	**1%**
Dietary Fiber 1g	**5%**
Sugars less than 1g	
Protein 2g	

Vitamin A 6%	•	Vitamin C 15%
Calcium 0%	•	Iron 2%

*Percent Daily Values are based on a 2,000 calorie diet

INGREDIENTS: CUT GREEN ASPARAGUS, WATER, SALT

Nutrition Facts

Serving Size 2 cookies (33g)
Servings Per Container about 10

Amount Per Serving

Calories 150 Calories from Fat 60

	% Daily Value*
Total Fat 6g	**9%**
Saturated Fat 3.5g	**10%**
Cholesterol 35mg	**11%**
Sodium 110mg	**8%**
Total Carbohydrate 22g	**7%**
Dietary Fiber less than 1g	**4%**
Sugars 9g	
Protein 2g	

Vitamin A 4%	•	Vitamin C 0%
Calcium 2%	•	Iron 5%

* Percent Daily Values are based on a 2,000 calorie diet. Your daily values may be higher or lower depending on your calorie needs.

		Calories	2000	2,500
Total Fat	Less than		65g	80g
Sat. Fat	Less than		20g	25g
Cholesterol	Less than		300mg	300mg
Sodium	Less than		2,400mg	2,400mg
Total Carbohydrate			300g	375g
Dietary Fiber			25g	30g

Calories per gram:
Fat 9 • Carbohydrate 4 • Protein 4

INGREDIENTS: BUTTER, BLEACHED ENRICHED WHEAT FLOUR [CONTAINS BLEACHED WHEAT FLOUR, WHEAT FLOUR, NIACIN, REDUCED IRON, THIAMINE (VITAMIN B₁), MONONITRATES, RIBOFLAVIN (VITAMIN B₂), FOLIC ACID]; ROLLED OATS, SUGAR, FANCY MOLASSES, BROWN SUGAR, MILK, LEAVENING (BAKING POWDER, BAKING SODA); SALT, NATURAL FLAVOR

vice size is for that food. If the label indicates one-half cup and you normally eat one full cup, you are consuming double the amount of fat, sugar, etc. on the label.

Calories are a characteristic of each basic food source. There are approximately nine calories per gram of fat, seven calories per gram of alcohol, four calories per gram of carbohydrate, and four calories per gram of protein. Obviously, foods with a higher fat content per serving will have more calories than an equal amount of a carbohydrate or protein. Remember, calories are simply calculated from the basic components of the food product and do not indicate the importance of the following nutritional information.

Total fats are an important component of many food products. With the exception of meats, milk, and oils, fat grams should be very low—approximately one to three grams per serving. Lean, trimmed meats should have no more than five grams of fat per serving. Low-fat cheese should have no more than one to two grams of fat per serving. Two-percent milk should have slightly less than five grams per eight-ounce glass. Products with a normally high fat content, such as cooking oils, may contain as much as seven to nine grams of fat, but the largest percentage of this fat should be poly- or monounsaturated. These are the so-called good fats.

Many products contain trans-fats, which are vegetable oils to which additional hydrogen ions have been added during preparation. Trans-fats have similar effects on our bodies as saturated animal fats and, when possible, should always be avoided. New federal guidelines on nutritional information will require that trans-fats be listed on nutritional labels by 2006.

Trying to reduce your intake of unnecessary fats, especially saturated fats, is good, healthy, and recommended on *Sugar Busters!* However, we do need some fat for the proper functioning of our bodies. Removing all fat from your diet is not healthy. When it comes to fat, remember moderation. Equally as harmful to us as foods with too much fat are those that are advertised as low or no fat, which usually means higher in sugar. Excessive amounts of added refined sugar will ultimately be converted to and stored in our bodies as fat.

Carbohydrates basically refer to all the sugar, either naturally occurring or added, in a particular food product. Fruits have a high content of fruit sugar (fructose), and milk products have a high content of milk sugar (lactose), but most carbohydrates are in the form of grains or starches and, as such, have very little simple sugars or "sugars." With the exception of fruits and dairy products, carbohydrate products, including grains and cereals, should contain no more than three grams of "sugars" per serving. A high "sugars" content—except in fruits and milk—is an important warning sign that the product is unacceptable on *Sugar Busters!* and probably has too much added refined sugar. Any increase in serving size can get you beyond the sugar limit very quickly.

Fiber is an extremely important component of many carbohydrates. The higher the fiber content of a food product, the healthier it is for you. The incidence of colon cancer as well as some other medical problems is greatly reduced in those people eating a high-fiber diet. You should eat at least twenty-five grams of fiber daily. Whole-grain products and green leafy vegetables are an excellent source of your daily fiber requirements.

Proteins may be derived from either plant or animal sources. Most of your protein will come from meat and dairy products, but grains and vegetables are also a good source. All balanced diets contain sufficient protein for your basic daily requirements.

Cholesterol is a component of most all meat

and dairy products. You should avoid ingesting unnecessary cholesterol, but, in most people, diets containing several hundred milligrams of cholesterol a day are not harmful. Only forty percent of the ingested cholesterol is actually absorbed into our systems. But, when given a choice of different foods in a particular category, choose the ones with the lowest cholesterol content.

Vitamins and minerals are both important to the proper functioning of our bodies. A well-balanced diet as suggested by the authors of *Sugar Busters!* contains all the essential vitamins and minerals. A glass of freshly squeezed orange or grapefruit juice contains as much potassium as a banana. Most foods contain more than an adequate amount of *sodium*. You should be careful about adding additional salt when cooking or seasoning, especially if you have a heart or blood pressure problem. If you do not eat a varied or balanced diet and are concerned about your daily intake of sufficient vitamins and minerals, a good commercially available vitamin with minerals, such as Theragran-M and Centrum, more than ensures adequate daily intake of these substances.

Other ingredients are supplements and additives that processors have included in the preparation of their food products. These can include unwanted glycemic ingredients like maltodextrin, dextrose, xylol, maltose, malt, isomalt, sugar alcohol, high-fructose corn syrup, hydrolyzed starch, hydrolyzed rice starch, enriched flour, syrups, honey, and brown sugar. On the label, they are listed in order, from the largest to the smallest amount. Although some of these terms are not familiar to you, they all are disguised sugars. They have been added for the purpose of enhancing the taste or thickening the particular product. Their ultimate effect will be to raise your insulin levels and create more fat on your body. Sugar alcohols, which are often present in low-sugar diet ice creams or candies, may cause gastrointestinal irritation and diarrhea. Although it is often difficult to avoid these additives altogether, every effort should be made to select those products that have as few and as little of these supplements as possible. Try to hold the total sugar alcohol consumption to less than 10 grams.

The category you need to pay particular attention to is total fats, which should not exceed one to three grams per serving except in meat and milk products (which should not exceed five grams per serving) and cooking oils (which should predominantly be poly- or monounsaturated fats). Total carbohydrates should generally be between fifteen and twenty-five grams per serving, with sugars not to exceed three grams per serving except in fruit and dairy products. Remember to pick the product in the particular food category with the highest fiber content. This also applies to cholesterol, where those products in a particular food category with the lowest amount of total cholesterol are preferable. The healthiest eating can be achieved by selecting stone ground or whole grains, fresh vegetables, and fruits. Cookies, cakes, pies, and most other low-fat and low-calorie items are full of the dreaded insulin-stimulating ingredients.

Regarding misleading titles or ingredient descriptions, a bread titled "Brand X" whole wheat bread may contain only a moderate amount of whole wheat unless it says 100 percent whole wheat or the only flour listed under "ingredients" is whole wheat flour. Try to buy only 100 percent whole grain or whole wheat breads. Now that *Sugar Busters!* has helped the nation see the huge problems (pun intended) associated with refined sugar and high-glycemic carbohydrate consumption, manufacturers, in the ingredients lists, are now calling their added sugar "natural cane crystals" or "dehydrated cane crystals." Are they concerned about your health? Certainly all of them are not!

Reading Labels

In summary, interpreting nutritional facts on food-product labels is not easy, but having a little knowledge about what this information means can make your shopping on *Sugar Busters!* much more successful.

Your Personal
Shopping List

As you become familiar with the acceptable brand-name products in your particular region of the country, add them to this guide to help you accomplish your grocery shopping more easily and quickly.

Your Personal Shopping List

Vegetables	Fruits
_____	_____
_____	_____
_____	_____
_____	_____
_____	_____
_____	_____
_____	_____
_____	_____
_____	_____
_____	_____
_____	_____
_____	_____

Your Personal Shopping List

Meat   Dairy

_____   _____

_____   _____

_____   _____

_____   _____

_____   _____

_____   _____

_____   _____

_____   _____

_____   _____

_____   _____

_____   _____

_____   _____

Seafood

Deli

_____ _____

_____ _____

_____ _____

_____ _____

_____ _____

_____ _____

_____ _____

_____ _____

_____ _____

_____ _____

_____ _____

_____ _____

Your Personal Shopping List

Bakery/Breads	Beverages
_____	_____
_____	_____
_____	_____
_____	_____
_____	_____
_____	_____
_____	_____
_____	_____
_____	_____
_____	_____
_____	_____
_____	_____

Your Personal Shopping List

Snacks & Crackers   Nuts & Seeds

_____   _____

_____   _____

_____   _____

_____   _____

_____   _____

_____   _____

_____   _____

_____   _____

_____   _____

_____   _____

_____   _____

Beans   Cereal (Cold/Hot)

————————————   ————————————

————————————   ————————————

————————————   ————————————

————————————   ————————————

————————————   ————————————

————————————   ————————————

————————————   ————————————

————————————   ————————————

————————————   ————————————

————————————   ————————————

————————————   ————————————

————————————   ————————————

Pancake Mixes/Flour Jams/Jellies

_____ _____

_____ _____

_____ _____

_____ _____

_____ _____

_____ _____

_____ _____

_____ _____

_____ _____

_____ _____

_____ _____

_____ _____

Your Personal Shopping List

Peanut Butter	Cocoa/Chocolate
_____	_____
_____	_____
_____	_____
_____	_____
_____	_____
_____	_____
_____	_____
_____	_____
_____	_____
_____	_____
_____	_____
_____	_____

Your Personal Shopping List

Tea/Coffee   Juice

_____   _____

_____   _____

_____   _____

_____   _____

_____   _____

_____   _____

_____   _____

_____   _____

_____   _____

_____   _____

_____   _____

Your Personal Shopping List

Soup (Dry/   Canned Meat/Fish
Canned)

_____   _____

_____   _____

_____   _____

_____   _____

_____   _____

_____   _____

_____   _____

_____   _____

_____   _____

_____   _____

_____   _____

Olives/Pickles/Garnishes/Condiments

_____

_____

_____

_____

_____

_____

_____

_____

_____

_____

_____

Your Personal Shopping List

Canned Fruit	Canned Vegetables
_____	_____
_____	_____
_____	_____
_____	_____
_____	_____
_____	_____
_____	_____
_____	_____
_____	_____
_____	_____
_____	_____
_____	_____

Your Personal Shopping List

Salad Dressings	Spaghetti Sauce
_____	_____
_____	_____
_____	_____
_____	_____
_____	_____
_____	_____
_____	_____
_____	_____
_____	_____
_____	_____
_____	_____
_____	_____

Your Personal Shopping List

Pasta

Gravy

_____   _____

_____   _____

_____   _____

_____   _____

_____   _____

_____   _____

_____   _____

_____   _____

_____   _____

_____   _____

_____   _____

_____   _____

Your Personal Shopping List

Box Dinners/
Prepared Foods

Ethnic/
Specialty Foods

_____   _____

_____   _____

_____   _____

_____   _____

_____   _____

_____   _____

_____   _____

_____   _____

_____   _____

_____   _____

Rice   Spices

_____   _____

_____   _____

_____   _____

_____   _____

_____   _____

_____   _____

_____   _____

_____   _____

_____   _____

_____   _____

_____   _____

_____   _____

Your Personal Shopping List

Cooking Oil

Cake/Flour

Your Personal Shopping List

Ice Cream   Frozen Food

_____   _____

_____   _____

_____   _____

_____   _____

_____   _____

_____   _____

_____   _____

_____   _____

_____   _____

_____   _____

_____   _____

_____   _____

Your Personal Shopping List

Alcohol	Additional Items
_____	_____
_____	_____
_____	_____
_____	_____
_____	_____
_____	_____
_____	_____
_____	_____
_____	_____
_____	_____
_____	_____
_____	_____

You bought the SHOPPER'S GUIDE, *now get
the new-and-improved must-have book that
inspired it all!*

THE NEW
SUGAR BUSTERS!®

Cut Sugar to Trim Fat

by H. Leighton Steward, Morrison
C. Bethea, M.D., Sam S. Andrews,
M.D., and Luis A. Balart, M.D.

Completely revised and updated with:

- **NEW recipes**
- **NEW meal plans**
- **NEW research**
- **NEW foods to eat**
- **NEW FAQs**

Plus:
- Amazing testimonials
- Essential weight-loss and nutrition facts for women
- How SUGAR BUSTERS! fights diabetes
- A new introduction by the authors

Published by Ballantine Books
Now available wherever books are sold

A delicious collection of more than 150 simple-to-make recipes and menu ideas.

SUGAR BUSTERS!® QUICK & EASY COOKBOOK

by H. Leighton Steward, Morrison C. Bethea, M.D., Sam S. Andrews, M.D., and Luis A. Balart, M.D.

With this wonderful cookbook, the SUGAR BUSTERS!® eating program can easily become part of your daily routine. Forget counting calories, weighing your food, and trying to figure out those confusing charts and graphs. The *SUGAR BUSTERS!® QUICK & EASY COOKBOOK* makes preparing tasty, low-sugar or sugar-free fare a snap.

Published by Ballantine Books
Available wherever books are sold